This publication is intended to provide educational information for the reader on the covered subjects. It is not intended to take the place of personalized medical counseling, diagnosis, and treatment from a trained healthcare professional.

ISBN 978-1-998455-43-0 (Paperback)
ISBN 978-1-998455-44-7 (eBook)

Printed and bound in USA
Published by Loons Press

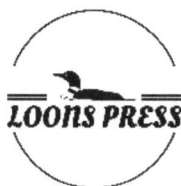

LOONS PRESS

Table Of Contents

How To Eliminate Gallstones Naturally

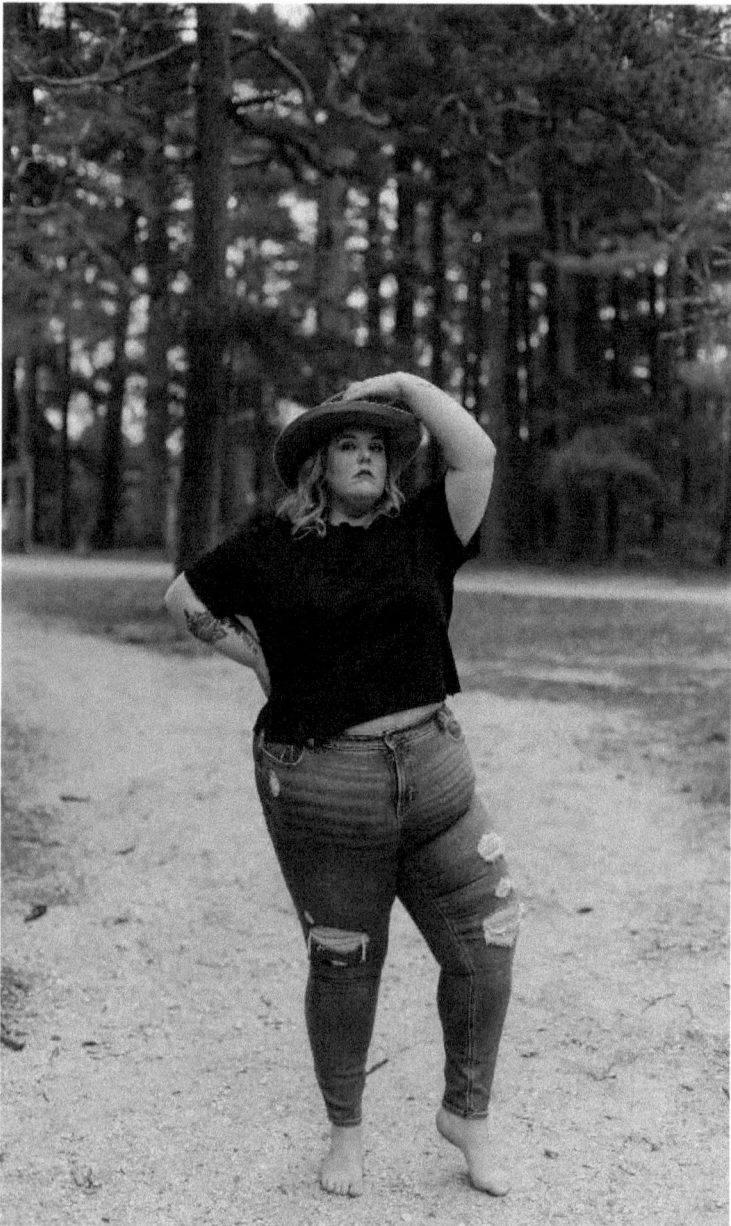

Chapter 1

Understanding Gallstones

What are Gallstones?

Gallstones are small, pebble-like substances that form in the gallbladder. They can vary in size, from as small as a grain of sand to as large as a golf ball. Gallstones are made up of cholesterol or bilirubin, a pigment produced by the liver. These stones can cause a variety of symptoms, including pain in the upper abdomen, back, or right shoulder blade, nausea, vomiting, and jaundice.

There are two main types of gallstones: cholesterol stones and pigment stones. Cholesterol stones are the most common type and are usually yellow-green in color. They are made up of hardened cholesterol and are often caused by an imbalance of bile salts or cholesterol in the bile. Pigment stones, on the other hand, are smaller and darker in color. They are made up of bilirubin and are often caused by conditions that affect the liver, such as cirrhosis or infections.

Gallstones can be diagnosed through various tests, including ultrasound, CT scans, and blood tests. Once diagnosed, treatment options may include medications to dissolve the stones, surgery to remove the gallbladder, or natural remedies to help pass the stones. It is important to consult with a healthcare provider to determine the best course of action for your specific situation.

If you are looking to eliminate gallstones naturally, there are several holistic approaches that may help. These may include dietary changes, such as increasing fiber intake and reducing saturated fats, as well as incorporating herbs and supplements that support gallbladder health. Physical activity, stress management techniques, and acupuncture may also be beneficial in promoting gallstone elimination.

Overall, understanding what gallstones are and how they form is essential in taking a proactive approach to managing and eliminating them. By adopting a holistic approach to recovery, you can work towards preventing future gallstones and promoting overall gallbladder health. Remember to consult with a healthcare provider before making any significant changes to your diet or lifestyle.

Types of Gallstones

In order to effectively eliminate gallstones naturally, it is important to understand the different types of gallstones that can form in the gallbladder. There are two main types of gallstones: cholesterol gallstones and pigment gallstones.

Cholesterol gallstones are the most common type of gallstones, accounting for about 80% of cases. These gallstones are primarily made up of cholesterol, which is a type of fat found in the bile. When there is an imbalance in the composition of bile, with too much cholesterol and not enough bile salts, cholesterol gallstones can form. These gallstones are usually yellow in color and can vary in size.

Pigment gallstones, on the other hand, are less common and are typically made up of bilirubin, a waste product produced by the liver. These gallstones are usually dark brown or black in color and are more likely to occur in people with certain medical conditions, such as cirrhosis or hemolytic anemia.

In addition to cholesterol and pigment gallstones, there are also mixed gallstones, which contain a combination of cholesterol and bilirubin. These gallstones can vary in color and composition, making them more difficult to treat.

It is important to note that the type of gallstones a person has can impact the treatment options available. For example, cholesterol gallstones may respond well to dietary changes and natural remedies, while pigment gallstones may require more aggressive treatments, such as medication or surgery.

By understanding the different types of gallstones and how they form, individuals can take a more targeted approach to eliminating gallstones naturally and effectively.

It is important to consult with a healthcare provider before starting any treatment plan to ensure it is safe and appropriate for your specific situation.

Symptoms of Gallstones

If you are experiencing symptoms such as severe abdominal pain, nausea, vomiting, and jaundice, you may be suffering from gallstones. These small, hard particles that form in the gallbladder can cause a variety of uncomfortable symptoms that can significantly impact your quality of life.

It is important to recognize the signs of gallstones so that you can take steps to eliminate them and prevent further complications.

One of the most common symptoms of gallstones is intense pain in the upper right side of the abdomen. This pain may come and go, but it is often triggered by eating fatty foods. The pain can be sharp or dull and may radiate to the back or shoulder.

If you are experiencing persistent abdominal pain, it is important to consult with a healthcare professional to determine if gallstones are the cause.

In addition to abdominal pain, gallstones can also cause nausea and vomiting. These symptoms may occur after eating a large or fatty meal and can be accompanied by bloating and indigestion. If you are experiencing frequent bouts of nausea and vomiting, it is important to seek medical attention to determine the underlying cause and develop a treatment plan.

Jaundice, a yellowing of the skin and eyes, can also be a sign of gallstones. This occurs when the bile ducts become blocked by gallstones, preventing the flow of bile from the liver to the intestines. Jaundice can also cause dark urine and pale stools. If you notice any changes in the color of your skin or eyes, it is important to consult with a healthcare professional to determine the cause and receive appropriate treatment.

Other symptoms of gallstones may include fever, chills, and a feeling of fullness in the abdomen. These symptoms can vary in severity and may come and go over time. If you are experiencing any of these symptoms, it is important to seek medical attention to determine if gallstones are the cause and to explore natural treatment options for eliminating them.

By recognizing the symptoms of gallstones and taking proactive steps to address them, you can improve your overall health and well-being.

How To Eliminate Gallstones Naturally

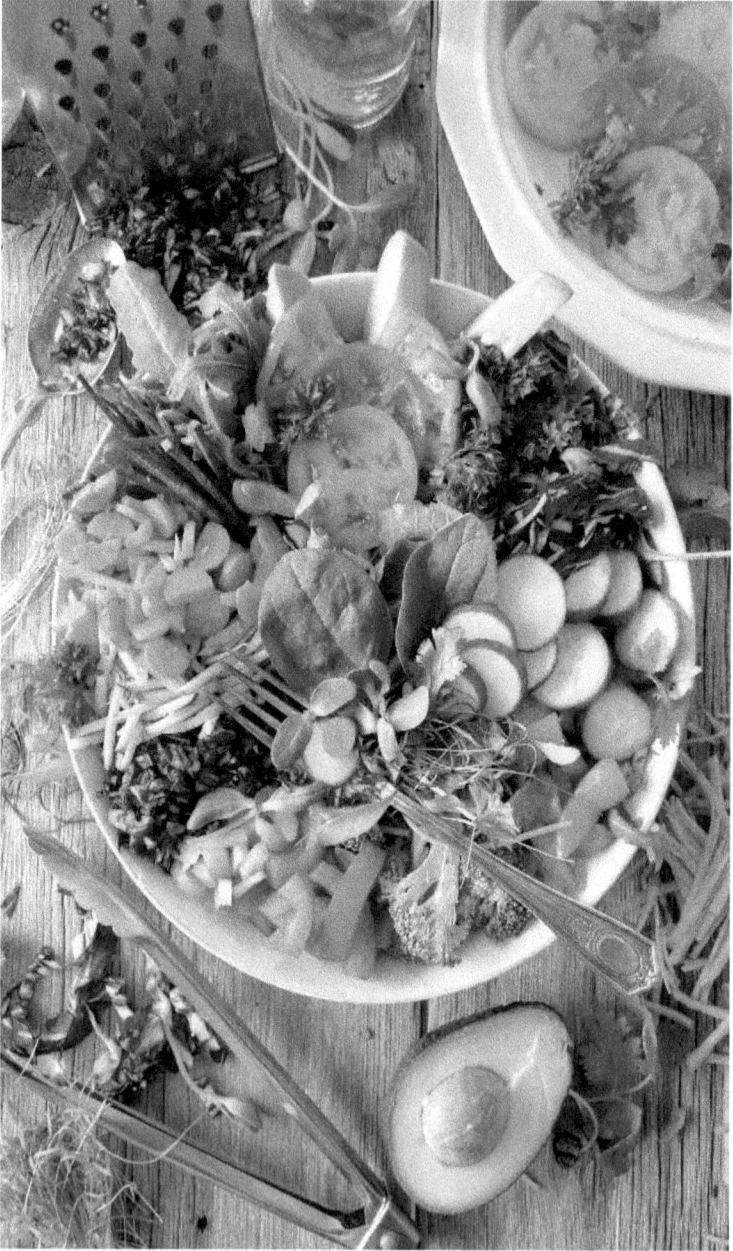

Chapter 2

Causes of Gallstones

Risk Factors for Gallstones

Gallstones are a common health issue that can cause severe pain and discomfort for those who suffer from them. There are several risk factors that can increase the likelihood of developing gallstones, and it's important for individuals to be aware of these factors in order to take preventative measures. One of the main risk factors for gallstones is being overweight or obese. Excess body fat can lead to an increased production of cholesterol in the liver, which can contribute to the formation of gallstones.

Another risk factor for gallstones is a diet high in fat and cholesterol. Consuming foods that are high in these substances can lead to an excess of cholesterol in the bile, which can then form into gallstones. It's important for individuals with gallstones to avoid foods that are high in fat and cholesterol in order to prevent further complications.

Additionally, a diet that is low in fiber can also increase the risk of developing gallstones. Fiber helps to regulate the digestive system and can help to prevent the buildup of cholesterol in the bile.

Other risk factors for gallstones include being female, over the age of 40, and having a family history of gallstones. Women are more likely than men to develop gallstones, especially those who have had multiple pregnancies or are taking hormone replacement therapy. Individuals over the age of 40 are also at a higher risk of developing gallstones, as the body's ability to break down cholesterol decreases with age.

Those with a family history of gallstones should be especially vigilant about their diet and lifestyle choices in order to prevent the formation of gallstones.

Certain medical conditions, such as diabetes and liver disease, can also increase the risk of developing gallstones. Individuals with these conditions should work closely with their healthcare provider to manage their symptoms and reduce their risk of developing gallstones.

Additionally, rapid weight loss or weight cycling can increase the risk of gallstones, as the body may release excess cholesterol into the bile during these periods of rapid change. It's important for individuals to focus on gradual, sustainable weight loss in order to reduce their risk of developing gallstones.

In order to prevent the formation of gallstones and reduce the risk of complications, individuals with gallstones should focus on maintaining a healthy diet, staying active, and managing any underlying medical conditions. By taking a proactive approach to their health and making positive lifestyle changes, individuals can reduce their risk of developing gallstones and improve their overall well-being.

It's important for those with gallstones to work closely with their healthcare provider to create a personalized plan for managing their condition and preventing future issues related to gallstones.

Medical Conditions that Increase Gallstone Formation

If you have been diagnosed with gallstones, you may be wondering what caused them to form in the first place. One of the factors that can contribute to the formation of gallstones is certain medical conditions. Understanding these conditions can help you take steps to prevent future gallstone formation and promote overall gallbladder health.

One medical condition that can increase the risk of gallstone formation is obesity. Excess body weight can lead to an imbalance in bile production and secretion, which can result in the formation of gallstones. If you are overweight or obese, it is important to work towards achieving a healthy weight through diet and exercise to reduce your risk of developing gallstones.

Another medical condition that is associated with an increased risk of gallstones is diabetes. People with diabetes are more likely to have high levels of triglycerides in their blood, which can contribute to the formation of gallstones.

Managing your blood sugar levels through diet, exercise, and medication can help reduce your risk of developing gallstones.

Liver disease is another medical condition that can lead to an increased risk of gallstone formation. Conditions such as cirrhosis or hepatitis can affect the production and secretion of bile, increasing the likelihood of gallstone formation. If you have liver disease, it is important to work closely with your healthcare provider to manage your condition and reduce your risk of developing gallstones.

Inflammatory bowel disease (IBD), such as Crohn's disease or ulcerative colitis, is also associated with an increased risk of gallstones. The inflammation and damage to the intestines that occur with these conditions can disrupt the normal function of the gallbladder and lead to the formation of gallstones. Managing your IBD symptoms and working with your healthcare provider to address any gastrointestinal issues can help reduce your risk of developing gallstones.

Overall, understanding the medical conditions that can increase the risk of gallstone formation can help you take proactive steps to protect your gallbladder health. By managing these conditions and making healthy lifestyle choices, you can reduce your risk of developing gallstones and promote overall well-being.

Remember to consult with your healthcare provider for personalized recommendations and treatment options tailored to your specific needs.

Lifestyle Factors Contributing to Gallstones

Gallstones are a common health issue that can cause discomfort and pain for those who suffer from them. While there are many factors that can contribute to the formation of gallstones, lifestyle choices play a significant role in their development.

By understanding and addressing these lifestyle factors, individuals can take proactive steps towards eliminating gallstones naturally and improving their overall health.

One lifestyle factor that can contribute to the formation of gallstones is diet. Consuming a diet high in saturated fats, cholesterol, and processed foods can increase the risk of developing gallstones.

To reduce this risk, individuals should focus on eating a diet rich in fruits, vegetables, whole grains, and lean proteins. Incorporating foods that are high in fiber and low in unhealthy fats can help to promote healthy digestion and prevent the formation of gallstones.

In addition to diet, maintaining a healthy weight is also important in preventing gallstones. Being overweight or obese can increase the risk of developing gallstones, as excess body fat can lead to an imbalance in cholesterol levels and impair the function of the gallbladder.

By engaging in regular physical activity and making healthy food choices, individuals can work towards achieving and maintaining a healthy weight, reducing their risk of developing gallstones.

Another lifestyle factor that can contribute to gallstone formation is dehydration. Inadequate water intake can lead to the concentration of bile in the gallbladder, increasing the likelihood of gallstone formation. Staying properly hydrated by drinking plenty of water throughout the day can help to prevent the development of gallstones and promote overall gallbladder health.

Stress is also a lifestyle factor that can impact the formation of gallstones. Chronic stress can lead to the release of cortisol, a hormone that can disrupt the balance of cholesterol in the body and contribute to the formation of gallstones.

Managing stress through relaxation techniques such as meditation, deep breathing, and yoga can help to reduce the risk of developing gallstones and promote overall well-being.

By addressing lifestyle factors such as diet, weight, hydration, and stress, individuals can take proactive steps towards eliminating gallstones naturally and improving their overall health.

Making positive changes in these areas can not only help to prevent the formation of gallstones but also promote overall well-being and vitality. By taking a holistic approach to recovery, individuals can work towards eliminating gallstones and achieving optimal health and wellness.

How To Eliminate Gallstones Naturally

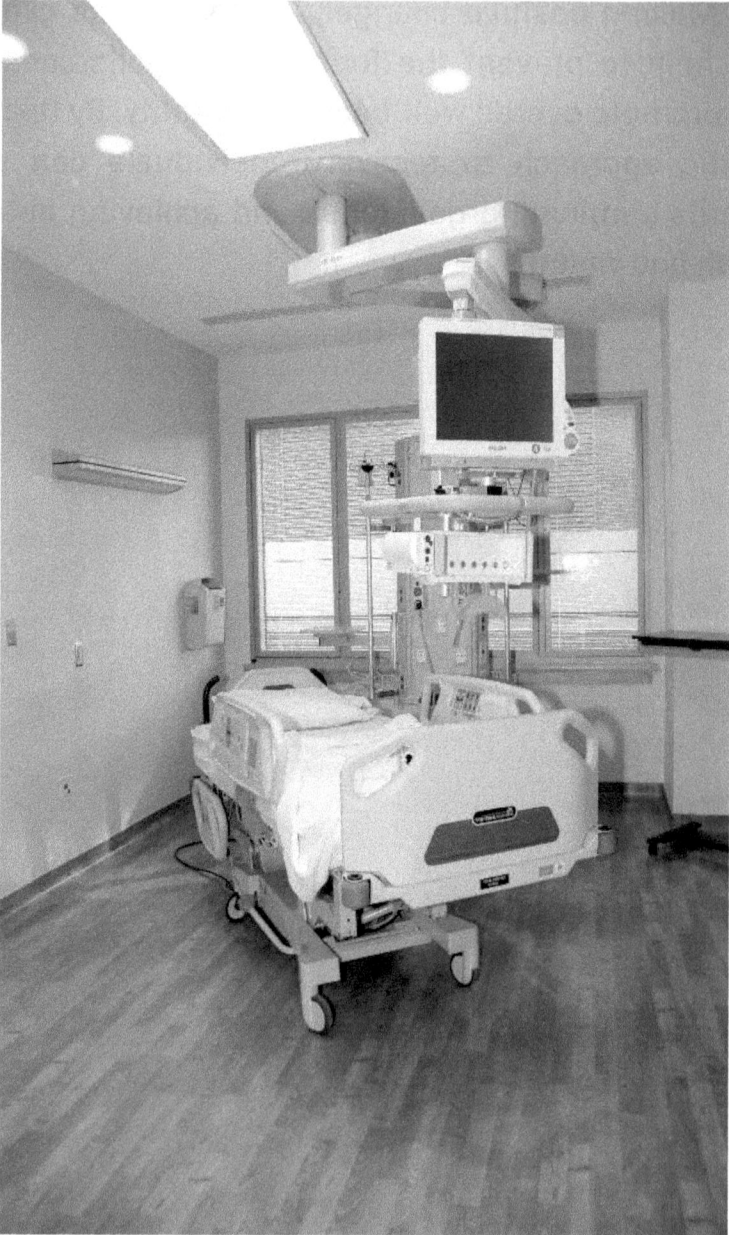

Chapter 3

Traditional Treatment Options for Gallstones

Medical Procedures for Gallstone Removal

If you have been diagnosed with gallstones, you may be wondering about the various medical procedures available for their removal. In this subchapter, we will explore some of the most common medical procedures used to eliminate gallstones and alleviate the associated symptoms. While natural remedies can be effective for some individuals, medical intervention may be necessary in more severe cases.

One of the most common medical procedures for gallstone removal is known as a cholecystectomy. This surgical procedure involves the removal of the gallbladder, the organ responsible for storing bile produced by the liver. While the gallbladder is not essential for survival, its removal can help prevent future gallstone formation and alleviate symptoms such as abdominal pain, nausea, and bloating.

Another common medical procedure for gallstone removal is known as an endoscopic retrograde cholangiopancreatography (ERCP). This procedure involves the insertion of a thin, flexible tube with a camera attached through the mouth and into the digestive tract. Once inside, the doctor can locate and remove gallstones from the bile ducts using specialized tools. ERCP is often used in cases where gallstones have migrated from the gallbladder to the bile ducts.

In some cases, medications may be prescribed to help dissolve gallstones. Ursodiol is a common medication used for this purpose, as it can help break down cholesterol-based gallstones over time. While medication may be effective for some individuals, it is not always successful in eliminating gallstones completely. In cases where medication is not effective, surgical intervention may be necessary.

Lithotripsy is another medical procedure used for gallstone removal. This non-invasive procedure involves the use of shock waves to break up gallstones into smaller pieces, making them easier to pass through the bile ducts.

While lithotripsy is less invasive than surgery, it may not be suitable for all individuals and is typically reserved for smaller gallstones.

It is important to consult with a healthcare provider to determine the most appropriate medical procedure for your individual situation. While natural remedies can be effective for some individuals, medical intervention may be necessary in more severe cases of gallstone formation. By understanding the various medical procedures available for gallstone removal, you can make an informed decision about the best course of action for your health and well-being.

Medications for Gallstone Dissolution

If you have been diagnosed with gallstones, you may be wondering what your treatment options are. One method for eliminating gallstones is through the use of medications designed to dissolve them. This subchapter will explore the various medications available for gallstone dissolution and how they can help you on your journey to recovery.

One common medication used for gallstone dissolution is Ursodiol, also known as ursodeoxycholic acid. This medication works by reducing the amount of cholesterol produced by the liver, which in turn helps to dissolve cholesterol-based gallstones. Ursodiol is typically taken in pill form and is often prescribed by doctors as a first-line treatment for mild to moderate gallstones.

Another medication that may be prescribed for gallstone dissolution is Chenodiol, also known as chenodeoxycholic acid. Chenodiol works in a similar way to Ursodiol by reducing cholesterol production in the liver. This medication is typically used for patients who are unable to tolerate Ursodiol or who do not respond to Ursodiol treatment.

In some cases, healthcare providers may recommend a combination of medications for gallstone dissolution. This combination therapy may include Ursodiol or Chenodiol along with other medications to help break down and eliminate gallstones. It is important to follow your healthcare provider's instructions carefully when taking these medications to ensure they are effective in dissolving your gallstones.

While medications can be effective for gallstone dissolution, it is important to remember that they are not a quick fix and may take several months to work. Additionally, medications may not be suitable for everyone, particularly those with severe gallstones or other underlying health conditions.

It is always best to consult with your healthcare provider to determine the best course of treatment for your specific situation.

Potential Side Effects of Traditional Treatments

If you are considering traditional treatments for gallstones, it is important to be aware of the potential side effects that may come with them. While these treatments can be effective in eliminating gallstones, they also carry risks and may not be the best option for everyone.

In this subchapter, we will explore some of the potential side effects of traditional treatments for gallstones.

One common traditional treatment for gallstones is surgery, specifically a cholecystectomy, which is the removal of the gallbladder. While this procedure is generally safe and effective, it is not without risks. Some potential side effects of cholecystectomy include infection, bleeding, and damage to surrounding organs.

Additionally, some people may experience digestive issues or diarrhea after having their gallbladder removed.

Another traditional treatment for gallstones is medication, such as ursodeoxycholic acid (UDCA) or chenodeoxycholic acid (CDCA). While these medications can help dissolve gallstones, they can also cause side effects such as diarrhea, nausea, and abdominal pain.

In rare cases, these medications can also cause liver damage. It is important to discuss the potential risks and benefits of medication with your healthcare provider before starting treatment.

Extracorporeal shock wave lithotripsy (ESWL) is another traditional treatment for gallstones that uses shock waves to break up the stones. While this treatment is non-invasive and generally safe, it can cause side effects such as abdominal pain, bruising, and pancreatitis. Additionally, ESWL may not be effective for all types of gallstones, so it is important to consult with a healthcare provider to determine if this treatment is right for you.

In contrast to traditional treatments, there are natural and holistic approaches to eliminating gallstones that may be gentler on the body and have fewer side effects. These approaches include dietary changes, herbal supplements, and lifestyle modifications.

By addressing the root causes of gallstones and supporting the body's natural detoxification processes, these holistic treatments can help prevent the formation of new stones and support overall health and well-being. If you are interested in exploring natural alternatives to traditional treatments for gallstones, be sure to consult with a healthcare provider or holistic practitioner who is experienced in this area.

How To Eliminate Gallstones Naturally

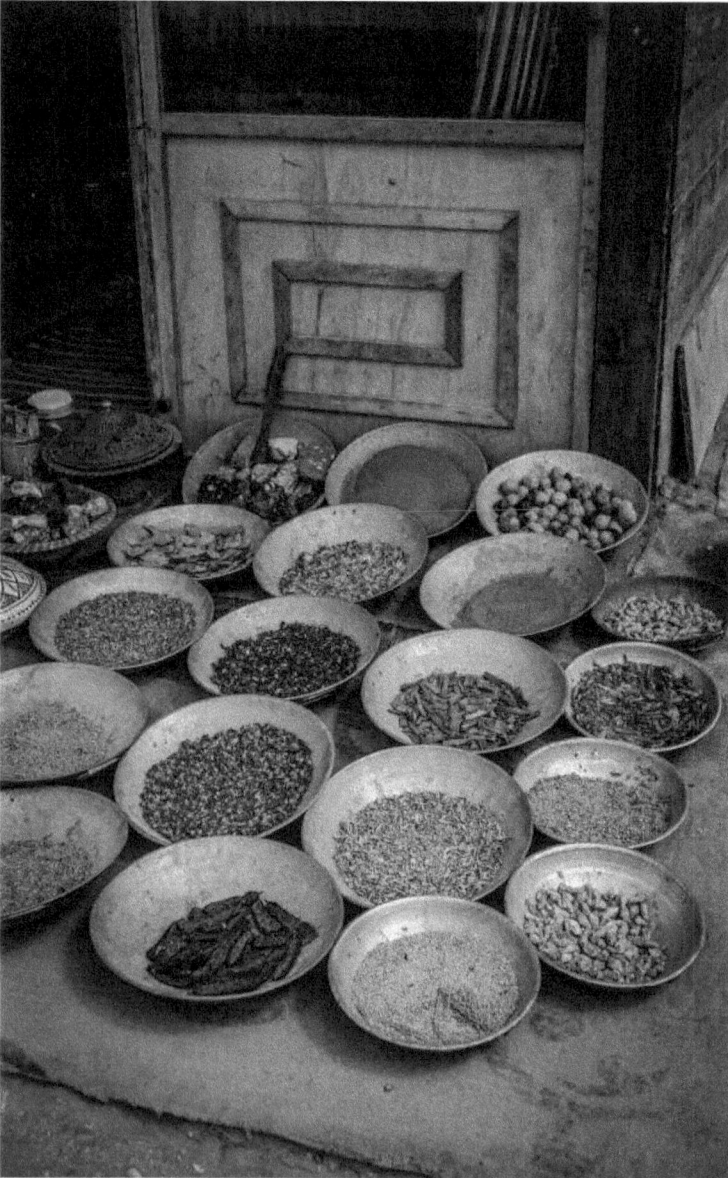

Chapter 4

Holistic Approaches to Gallstone Elimination

Dietary Changes for Gallstone Prevention

If you have been diagnosed with gallstones, making dietary changes is essential for preventing future episodes and promoting overall gallstone elimination. By focusing on a holistic approach to recovery, you can take control of your health and reduce the risk of complications associated with gallstones.

In this subchapter, we will explore some dietary changes that can help prevent the formation of gallstones and support your body's natural healing process.

How To Eliminate Gallstones Naturally

One of the most important dietary changes you can make for gallstone prevention is to increase your intake of fiber-rich foods. Fiber helps to regulate digestion and promote healthy bowel movements, which can prevent the build-up of cholesterol in the gallbladder.

Foods high in fiber include fruits, vegetables, whole grains, and legumes. By incorporating these foods into your diet, you can help to reduce the risk of developing new gallstones.

In addition to increasing your fiber intake, it is also important to limit your consumption of high-fat and processed foods. These types of foods can contribute to the build-up of cholesterol in the gallbladder, leading to the formation of gallstones. Instead, focus on eating a balanced diet that includes lean proteins, healthy fats, and plenty of fruits and vegetables.

By making these changes, you can support your body's natural detoxification process and reduce the risk of gallstone formation.

Another important dietary change for gallstone prevention is to stay hydrated. Drinking plenty of water helps to flush out toxins from the body and keep the digestive system running smoothly. Aim to drink at least eight glasses of water a day, and consider adding lemon or lime to your water for added benefits. By staying hydrated, you can help to prevent the build-up of cholesterol in the gallbladder and reduce the risk of developing new gallstones.

In conclusion, making dietary changes for gallstone prevention is an important step in promoting overall health and well-being. By increasing your fiber intake, limiting high-fat foods, and staying hydrated, you can support your body's natural healing process and reduce the risk of complications associated with gallstones.

Remember to consult with your healthcare provider before making any significant changes to your diet, and consider working with a holistic health practitioner to develop a personalized plan for gallstone elimination. By taking a proactive approach to your health, you can support your body in its natural healing process and prevent future episodes of gallstone formation.

Herbal Remedies for Gallstone Dissolution

In this subchapter, we will explore some of the most effective herbal remedies for dissolving gallstones naturally. These remedies have been used for centuries in traditional medicine and have shown promising results in helping to eliminate gallstones without the need for surgery or medication.

One of the most popular herbal remedies for gallstone dissolution is Chanca Piedra, also known as "stone breaker." This herb has been used in South American traditional medicine for generations to help break down kidney and gallstones. Studies have shown that Chanca Piedra can help to dissolve gallstones by reducing the amount of cholesterol in the bile, which is a major factor in the formation of gallstones.

Another powerful herb for gallstone dissolution is milk thistle. Milk thistle contains a compound called silymarin, which has been shown to have antioxidant and anti-inflammatory properties that can help to protect the liver and gallbladder.

By supporting liver function, milk thistle can help to improve bile flow and reduce the risk of gallstone formation.

Turmeric is another herb that has been used for centuries in traditional medicine for its anti-inflammatory and antioxidant properties. Studies have shown that turmeric can help to reduce inflammation in the gallbladder and improve bile flow, which can aid in the dissolution of gallstones. Adding turmeric to your diet or taking a turmeric supplement can be an effective way to support gallstone elimination.

Dandelion root is another herbal remedy that can help to support gallstone dissolution. Dandelion root contains compounds that can help to stimulate bile production and improve liver function, which can aid in the breakdown of gallstones. Dandelion root can be taken as a tea or supplement to help support the natural elimination of gallstones.

Incorporating these herbal remedies into your daily routine can help to support the natural dissolution of gallstones and promote overall gallbladder health.

However, it is important to speak with a healthcare provider before starting any new herbal remedies, especially if you are currently taking medication or have underlying health conditions. With the right combination of herbal remedies and lifestyle changes, you can take a holistic approach to eliminating gallstones naturally and improving your overall well-being.

Lifestyle Modifications to Support Gallstone Elimination

In order to effectively eliminate gallstones naturally, it is important to make certain lifestyle modifications that support the process. These modifications can help to prevent the formation of new gallstones and aid in the elimination of existing ones.

By incorporating these changes into your daily routine, you can support your body's natural ability to heal and recover from gallstones.

One key lifestyle modification to support gallstone elimination is to maintain a healthy diet. This means avoiding foods that are high in cholesterol and saturated fats, as these can contribute to the formation of gallstones. Instead, focus on eating a diet rich in fruits, vegetables, whole grains, and lean proteins. Incorporating foods that are high in fiber can also help to promote healthy digestion and reduce the risk of gallstone formation.

In addition to a healthy diet, regular exercise is another important lifestyle modification to support gallstone elimination. Physical activity can help to improve overall health and digestion, which can aid in the elimination of gallstones. Aim to incorporate at least 30 minutes of moderate exercise into your daily routine, such as walking, cycling, or swimming. Exercise not only supports gallstone elimination, but also helps to reduce stress and improve mood.

Staying hydrated is also crucial for supporting gallstone elimination. Drinking plenty of water throughout the day can help to flush out toxins and prevent the build-up of gallstones.

Aim to drink at least 8-10 glasses of water each day, and consider adding lemon or apple cider vinegar to your water to help support digestion and liver function. Staying hydrated can also help to reduce symptoms of gallstones, such as pain and discomfort.

Lastly, managing stress is an important lifestyle modification for supporting gallstone elimination. Chronic stress can have a negative impact on digestion and overall health, which can worsen symptoms of gallstones. Incorporate stress-reducing activities into your daily routine, such as meditation, yoga, or deep breathing exercises.

Prioritizing self-care and relaxation can help to support your body's natural healing process and aid in the elimination of gallstones. By making these lifestyle modifications, you can support your body in eliminating gallstones naturally and promoting overall health and well-being.

How To Eliminate Gallstones Naturally

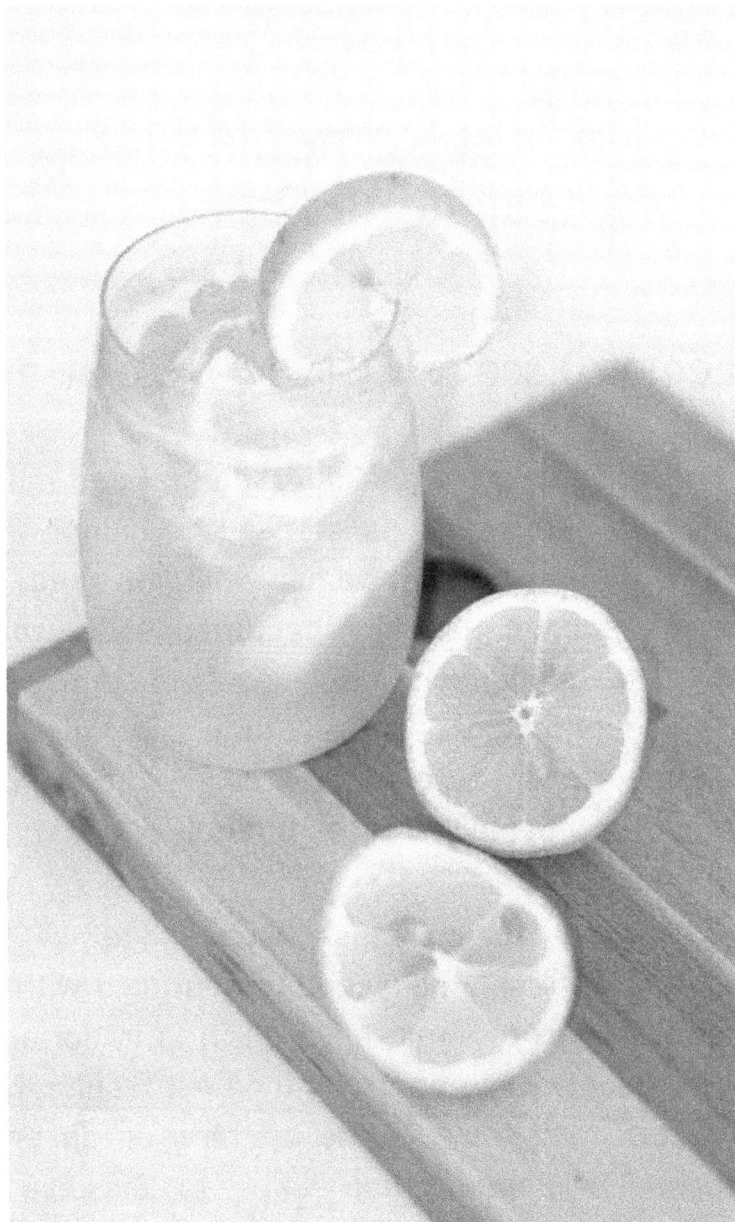

A Holistic Approach to Recovery

Chapter 5

Natural Remedies for Gallstone Relief

Lemon Juice and Olive Oil Cleanse

For those who are seeking a natural and holistic approach to eliminating gallstones, the Lemon Juice and Olive Oil Cleanse may be just what you need. This method has been used for centuries as a way to cleanse the gallbladder and liver, helping to break down and eliminate gallstones naturally. By following a few simple steps, you can potentially avoid the need for surgery or other invasive treatments.

To begin the cleanse, mix together one tablespoon of freshly squeezed lemon juice with one tablespoon of extra virgin olive oil. It is important to use high-quality ingredients for the best results. Drink this mixture first thing in the morning on an empty stomach. The lemon juice helps to dissolve the gallstones, while the olive oil helps to lubricate the gallbladder and facilitate their passage.

It is recommended to follow a strict diet during the cleanse to support the process of eliminating gallstones. Avoiding processed foods, fried foods, and dairy products is essential. Instead, focus on consuming plenty of fresh fruits and vegetables, whole grains, and lean proteins. Drinking plenty of water throughout the day is also important to help flush out toxins from the body.

During the Lemon Juice and Olive Oil Cleanse, you may experience some discomfort as the gallstones begin to pass through the bile ducts. This is normal and temporary. It is important to listen to your body and rest as needed during this time. Some individuals may also experience nausea or diarrhea, but these symptoms should subside as the cleanse progresses.

After completing the Lemon Juice and Olive Oil Cleanse, it is important to continue with a healthy diet and lifestyle to prevent the formation of new gallstones. Regular exercise, stress management, and maintaining a healthy weight are all important factors in preventing gallstones from reoccurring.

By taking a holistic approach to gallstone elimination, you can potentially avoid the need for surgery and improve your overall health and well-being.

Apple Cider Vinegar Treatment

If you are one of the many people who suffer from gallstones, you may be interested in exploring natural treatment options to help alleviate your symptoms and prevent future flare-ups. One such treatment that has gained popularity in recent years is apple cider vinegar. In this subchapter, we will discuss how apple cider vinegar can be used as a holistic approach to eliminating gallstones.

Apple cider vinegar is made from fermented apples and contains acetic acid, which has been shown to have numerous health benefits. One of the ways in which apple cider vinegar can help with gallstones is by breaking down the cholesterol that forms the stones. By incorporating apple cider vinegar into your daily routine, you may be able to help dissolve existing gallstones and prevent new ones from forming.

There are several ways in which you can incorporate apple cider vinegar into your treatment plan. One option is to mix a tablespoon of apple cider vinegar with a glass of water and drink it before each meal.

This can help stimulate bile production and aid in the digestion of fats, which can help prevent gallstones from forming. You can also add apple cider vinegar to your salads or use it as a marinade for meats and vegetables.

In addition to helping dissolve gallstones, apple cider vinegar can also help alleviate some of the symptoms associated with gallstone attacks. For example, the acetic acid in apple cider vinegar can help neutralize stomach acid, which can help reduce the pain and discomfort that often accompanies gallstone attacks.

By incorporating apple cider vinegar into your daily routine, you may be able to experience relief from your symptoms and improve your overall quality of life.

It is important to note that while apple cider vinegar can be a helpful tool in the treatment of gallstones, it is not a cure-all. It is always best to consult with a healthcare provider before starting any new treatment regimen, especially if you have a medical condition like gallstones. However, for many people, apple cider vinegar can be a valuable addition to a holistic approach to eliminating gallstones and improving overall health and well-being.

Turmeric and Ginger Tea for Gallstone Relief

If you are suffering from gallstones and looking for a natural remedy to help alleviate your symptoms, turmeric and ginger tea may be just what you need. These two powerful herbs have been used for centuries for their healing properties and can provide relief for those dealing with gallstone pain.

Turmeric is known for its anti-inflammatory and antioxidant properties, which can help reduce inflammation in the gallbladder and ease the pain associated with gallstones.

Ginger, on the other hand, is a natural pain reliever and can help soothe the digestive system, making it easier for your body to pass gallstones naturally.

To make turmeric and ginger tea, simply boil water and add a teaspoon of turmeric powder and a few slices of fresh ginger. Let the mixture steep for about 10 minutes, then strain and drink the tea while it is still warm. You can sweeten the tea with honey or lemon if desired.

Drinking turmeric and ginger tea regularly can help support your body's natural detoxification processes and may even help prevent the formation of new gallstones. It is important to note that while this tea can provide relief for some individuals, it is not a substitute for medical treatment. If you are experiencing severe gallstone symptoms, it is important to consult with a healthcare professional.

In conclusion, turmeric and ginger tea can be a valuable addition to your holistic approach to gallstone relief. By incorporating this natural remedy into your daily routine, you may find relief from pain and discomfort associated with gallstones.

How To Eliminate Gallstones Naturally

Remember to listen to your body and consult with a healthcare provider for personalized advice on managing your gallstone symptoms naturally.

How To Eliminate Gallstones Naturally

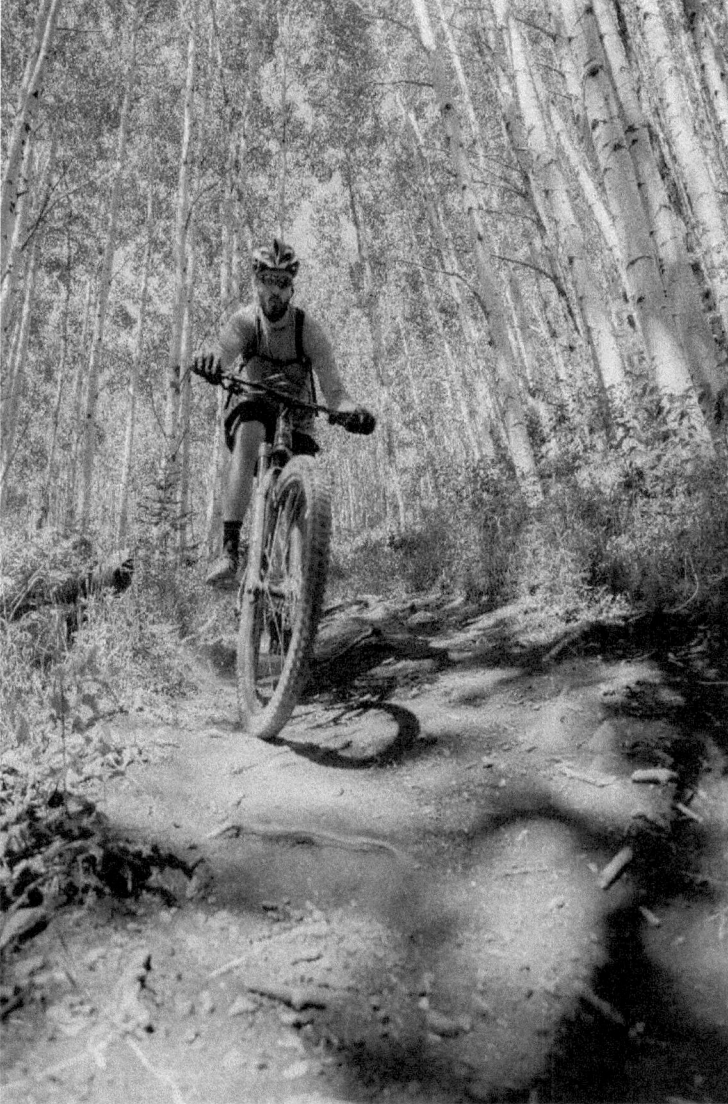

Chapter 6

Incorporating Holistic Practices into Daily Life

Stress Management Techniques for Gallstone Prevention

Gallstones can be a painful and frustrating condition to deal with, but there are ways to manage stress that can help prevent them from forming in the first place. Stress has been linked to an increase in gallstone formation, so finding effective stress management techniques is crucial for those looking to avoid this painful condition.

One effective stress management technique for preventing gallstones is deep breathing exercises. Taking deep, slow breaths can help relax the body and mind, reducing stress levels and promoting overall well-being. Practicing deep breathing exercises regularly can help keep stress at bay and reduce the risk of developing gallstones.

Another helpful stress management technique for gallstone prevention is regular exercise. Physical activity has been shown to reduce stress levels and improve overall health, which can in turn help prevent the formation of gallstones. Aim to incorporate at least 30 minutes of moderate exercise into your daily routine to keep stress levels in check and reduce your risk of developing gallstones.

Mindfulness meditation is another effective stress management technique for gallstone prevention. By focusing on the present moment and practicing mindfulness, you can reduce stress and anxiety levels, which can help prevent the formation of gallstones. Incorporating mindfulness meditation into your daily routine can help you stay calm and focused, reducing your risk of developing this painful condition.

In addition to these stress management techniques, it's important to maintain a healthy diet and lifestyle to prevent gallstones. Eating a diet rich in fruits, vegetables, and whole grains, and avoiding high-fat, processed foods can help reduce the risk of gallstone formation. Staying hydrated and getting an adequate amount of sleep each night are also important factors in preventing gallstones.

By incorporating these stress management techniques and healthy habits into your daily routine, you can reduce your risk of developing gallstones and promote overall well-being.

Exercise and Physical Activity Recommendations

Exercise and physical activity play a crucial role in the natural elimination of gallstones. In order to effectively break down and pass gallstones, it is important to stay active and maintain a healthy level of physical fitness. Regular exercise helps to improve digestion, reduce inflammation, and promote overall wellness, all of which are essential for gallstone elimination.

For individuals with gallstones, it is recommended to engage in a combination of cardiovascular exercise, strength training, and flexibility exercises. Cardiovascular exercise, such as walking, jogging, or cycling, helps to improve circulation and promote the flow of bile, which can aid in the breakdown of gallstones.

Strength training exercises, such as weightlifting or bodyweight exercises, help to increase muscle mass and improve metabolism, which can also support gallstone elimination.

In addition to cardiovascular and strength training exercises, flexibility exercises, such as yoga or stretching, can help to improve mobility and reduce the risk of gallstone-related complications. It is important to incorporate a variety of exercises into your routine in order to target different muscle groups and promote overall health and well-being.

It is recommended to aim for at least 30 minutes of moderate-intensity exercise most days of the week in order to support gallstone elimination. However, it is important to listen to your body and start slowly if you are new to exercise or recovering from a gallstone-related procedure.

Consult with a healthcare provider before starting any new exercise program, especially if you have existing health conditions.

Overall, incorporating regular exercise and physical activity into your daily routine is essential for natural gallstone elimination. By staying active and maintaining a healthy level of physical fitness, you can support the breakdown and elimination of gallstones, improve digestion, and promote overall wellness. Remember to consult with a healthcare provider before starting any new exercise program to ensure it is safe and appropriate for your individual needs.

Mindfulness and Meditation for Gallstone Recovery

Mindfulness and meditation are powerful tools that can greatly aid in the recovery process for those suffering from gallstones. By incorporating these practices into your daily routine, you can reduce stress, improve overall well-being, and support the body's natural healing processes.

When dealing with the pain and discomfort of gallstones, it is easy to become overwhelmed and stressed. Mindfulness practices, such as deep breathing exercises and guided meditation, can help calm the mind and body, reducing anxiety and increasing feelings of relaxation.

By learning to be present in the moment and focus on the breath, you can better cope with the challenges of gallstone recovery.

In addition to reducing stress, mindfulness and meditation can also help improve your overall health and well-being. Studies have shown that these practices can lower blood pressure, improve sleep quality, and boost the immune system. By taking the time to care for your mental and emotional health, you are supporting your body's ability to heal and recover from gallstones naturally.

Incorporating mindfulness and meditation into your daily routine can also help you better listen to your body's signals and respond to its needs. By tuning into your body's cues, you can better understand what triggers your gallstone symptoms and make positive lifestyle changes to support your recovery. By practicing mindfulness, you can cultivate a greater sense of self-awareness and make more informed choices about your health.

Overall, mindfulness and meditation are valuable tools for anyone looking to eliminate gallstones naturally. By reducing stress, improving overall well-being, and listening to your body's signals, you can support your body's natural healing processes and promote a faster recovery. By incorporating these practices into your daily routine, you can take a holistic approach to gallstone elimination and support your body in achieving optimal health and wellness.

How To Eliminate Gallstones Naturally

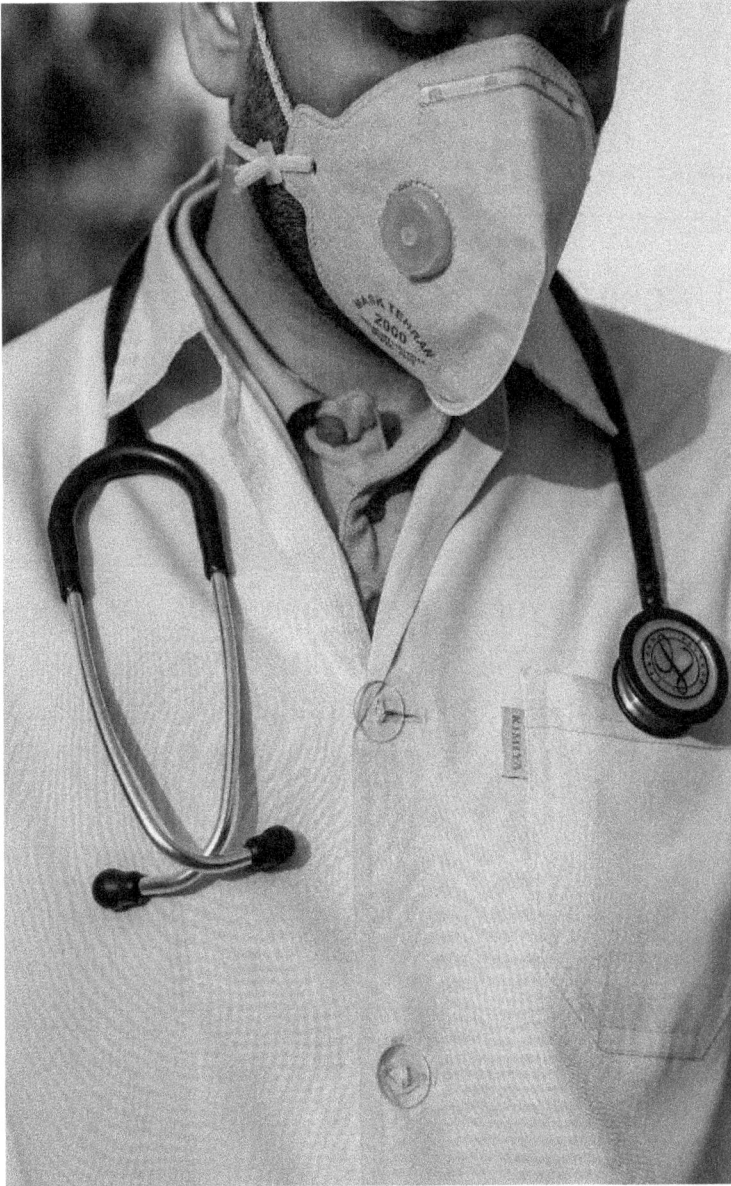

A Holistic Approach to Recovery

Chapter 7

Monitoring Gallstone Elimination Progress

Tracking Symptoms and Progress

Tracking symptoms and progress is an essential aspect of managing gallstones naturally. By keeping track of your symptoms, you can better understand what triggers flare-ups and make necessary adjustments to your lifestyle and diet. It is crucial to pay attention to any changes in your symptoms, such as increased pain, nausea, or digestive issues, as this can indicate the progression of gallstones or potential complications.

One way to track your symptoms is by keeping a journal or diary. Write down the date, time, and details of any symptoms you experience, as well as what you ate or did leading up to the flare-up. This can help you identify patterns and make connections between certain foods or activities and your symptoms.

By tracking your symptoms consistently, you can also monitor your progress and see if any changes you have made to your diet or lifestyle are having a positive impact on your gallstones.

Another important aspect of tracking symptoms and progress is keeping regular appointments with your healthcare provider. They can help monitor the size and number of your gallstones through imaging tests, such as ultrasounds, and provide guidance on the best course of action for managing your condition. Your healthcare provider can also offer advice on natural remedies and supplements that may help alleviate your symptoms and support gallstone elimination.

In addition to tracking your symptoms and progress, it is crucial to maintain a healthy lifestyle to support the natural elimination of gallstones. This includes eating a balanced diet rich in fruits, vegetables, whole grains, and lean proteins, as well as staying hydrated and engaging in regular physical activity. Avoiding trigger foods, such as fried and fatty foods, can also help reduce the likelihood of gallstone flare-ups.

Overall, tracking symptoms and progress is a vital part of managing gallstones naturally. By staying informed about your condition, making necessary lifestyle changes, and working closely with your healthcare provider, you can take control of your health and support the natural elimination of gallstones. Remember to be patient and consistent in your efforts, as natural remedies may take time to show results.

Consulting with Healthcare Providers

Consulting with healthcare providers is an essential step in the journey to eliminate gallstones naturally. While holistic approaches can be effective, it is important to consult with a healthcare provider to ensure that the chosen methods are safe and appropriate for individual needs.

Healthcare providers can offer valuable insights and guidance based on their knowledge and expertise, helping to create a personalized plan for eliminating gallstones.

When consulting with healthcare providers, it is important to be open and honest about your condition and any symptoms you may be experiencing. This information will help healthcare providers make an accurate diagnosis and recommend the most effective treatment options.

Additionally, discussing any previous medical history or conditions can help healthcare providers better understand your overall health and tailor their recommendations accordingly.

Healthcare providers can offer a range of treatment options for gallstone elimination, including dietary changes, supplements, and lifestyle modifications. They can also provide information on potential risks and side effects of different treatments, helping you make informed decisions about your healthcare.

By working closely with healthcare providers, you can develop a comprehensive plan that addresses the root causes of gallstones and promotes overall wellness.

In addition to providing treatment recommendations, healthcare providers can also offer support and encouragement throughout the gallstone elimination process. They can monitor your progress, answer any questions or concerns you may have, and make adjustments to your treatment plan as needed. Building a strong relationship with your healthcare provider can help you feel confident and empowered in your journey towards better health.

Overall, consulting with healthcare providers is a crucial step in the holistic approach to eliminating gallstones. By working together, you can develop a personalized plan that addresses your unique needs and promotes long-term health and wellness.

Remember to communicate openly with your healthcare provider, follow their recommendations closely, and stay committed to your treatment plan for the best results.

Adjusting Holistic Approaches as Needed

Adjusting holistic approaches as needed is a crucial aspect of effectively eliminating gallstones naturally. While following a holistic approach to recovery can be incredibly beneficial, it's important to remember that everyone's body is different. What works for one person may not work for another, so it's essential to be flexible and willing to make adjustments as needed.

One way to adjust your holistic approach is to pay attention to your body's response to the treatments you are using. If you find that a particular remedy or lifestyle change is not producing the desired results, it may be time to try something different.

It's important to listen to your body and trust your instincts when it comes to making adjustments to your holistic approach.

Another way to adjust your holistic approach is to seek guidance from a healthcare professional who specializes in natural remedies for gallstone elimination. They can provide valuable insight and personalized recommendations based on your unique situation.

Working with a professional can help you tailor your holistic approach to better suit your individual needs and optimize your chances of success.

In addition to seeking professional guidance, it's also helpful to do your own research and stay informed about the latest developments in natural remedies for gallstone elimination.

The more knowledge you have, the better equipped you will be to make informed decisions about adjusting your holistic approach as needed. Stay open-minded and willing to try new approaches that may benefit you on your journey to recovery.

Remember, the key to successfully eliminating gallstones naturally is to stay committed to your holistic approach and be willing to make adjustments as needed. By listening to your body, seeking guidance from professionals, and staying informed, you can optimize your chances of success and achieve a healthier, gallstone-free life. Adjusting holistic approaches as needed is a proactive step towards achieving your goal of natural gallstone elimination.

How To Eliminate Gallstones Naturally

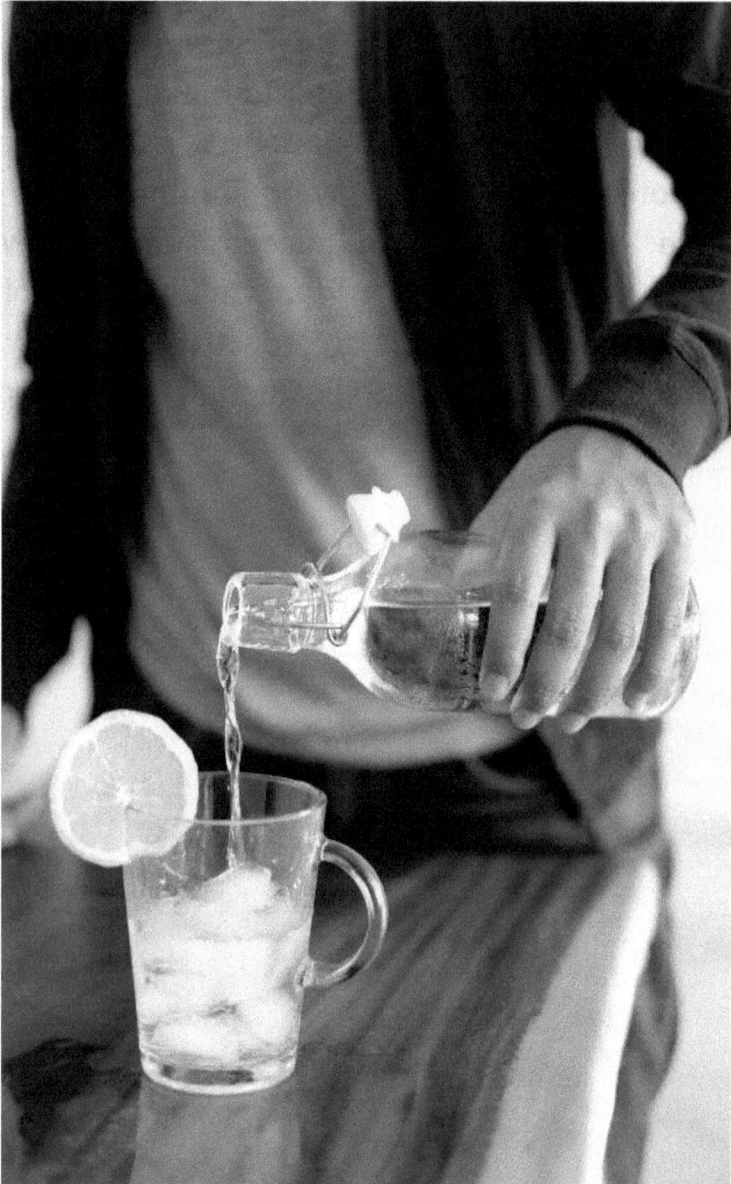

Chapter 8

Maintaining Gallstone-Free Health

Long-Term Strategies for Gallstone Prevention

Gallstones can be a painful and frustrating condition to deal with, but there are long-term strategies that can help prevent them from forming in the first place. By making some simple lifestyle changes and incorporating certain habits into your daily routine, you can significantly reduce your risk of developing gallstones in the future.

One of the most important long-term strategies for preventing gallstones is maintaining a healthy weight. Being overweight or obese can increase your risk of developing gallstones, so it's essential to focus on eating a balanced diet and getting regular exercise. By making healthy food choices and staying active, you can keep your weight in check and reduce your risk of gallstone formation.

Another key long-term strategy for preventing gallstones is to stay hydrated. Drinking plenty of water throughout the day can help keep your bile fluid diluted, which can prevent the formation of gallstones. Aim to drink at least eight glasses of water per day, and consider adding lemon or lime juice to your water for an extra boost of bile production.

In addition to maintaining a healthy weight and staying hydrated, incorporating foods into your diet that are high in fiber can also help prevent gallstones. Fiber-rich foods, such as fruits, vegetables, whole grains, and legumes, can help keep your digestive system running smoothly and prevent the buildup of cholesterol in your gallbladder. Aim to include a variety of fiber-rich foods in your meals each day to support gallstone prevention.

Lastly, reducing your intake of saturated fats and cholesterol can also help prevent gallstones from forming. Foods high in saturated fats and cholesterol can lead to an increase in cholesterol production in the liver, which can contribute to the formation of gallstones.

Focus on choosing lean proteins, such as poultry, fish, and beans, and opt for healthy fats, such as olive oil and avocado, to support gallstone prevention in the long term.

By incorporating these long-term strategies into your daily routine, you can reduce your risk of developing gallstones and support overall gallbladder health for years to come.

Recommended Check-Ups and Screenings

Regular check-ups and screenings are essential for individuals with gallstones to monitor their condition and ensure early detection of any complications.

It is recommended that individuals with gallstones undergo an annual physical exam to assess their overall health and well-being. During this exam, healthcare providers may perform blood tests to check for liver function and assess cholesterol levels, which can contribute to the formation of gallstones.

In addition to annual check-ups, individuals with gallstones should also consider scheduling regular ultrasounds to monitor the size and location of their gallstones. Ultrasounds can help healthcare providers determine if there are any changes in the gallbladder or surrounding organs that may require further investigation.

It is important to work closely with your healthcare provider to establish a screening schedule that is tailored to your individual needs and risk factors.

For individuals who have a history of gallstones or are at increased risk for developing them, additional screenings may be recommended. These screenings may include a gallbladder function test, also known as a hepatobiliary iminodiacetic acid (HIDA) scan, which can assess how well the gallbladder is functioning and identify any blockages in the bile ducts.

Other tests, such as a computed tomography (CT) scan or magnetic resonance imaging (MRI), may be recommended if there are concerns about complications such as inflammation or infection.

In some cases, healthcare providers may recommend more frequent screenings or additional tests based on individual risk factors. For example, individuals who have a family history of gallstones or certain medical conditions such as diabetes may require more frequent monitoring.

It is important to communicate openly with your healthcare provider about any concerns or changes in your symptoms to ensure that you are receiving the appropriate screenings and care.

By staying proactive about your health and following recommended check-ups and screenings, individuals with gallstones can better manage their condition and reduce the risk of complications. Remember, early detection is key to successful treatment and recovery.

Work closely with your healthcare provider to establish a personalized screening schedule that meets your individual needs and helps you maintain optimal health and well-being.

Support Systems for Gallstone Recovery

Support systems are crucial for individuals going through the process of recovering from gallstones. Whether you are opting for a holistic approach or traditional medical treatment, having a strong support system can make a significant difference in your recovery journey.

Here are some key support systems to consider as you navigate the process of eliminating gallstones naturally.

1. Family and Friends: Surround yourself with loved ones who understand your condition and are there to offer emotional support. Family and friends can provide encouragement, help with daily tasks, and be a source of comfort during challenging times. Having a strong support system of people who care about your well-being can make a world of difference in your recovery process.

2. Healthcare Professionals: It is essential to have a team of healthcare professionals who are knowledgeable about gallstone elimination and can provide guidance and support throughout your recovery journey. This may include a primary care physician, a gastroenterologist, a nutritionist, and other specialists who can offer valuable insights and recommendations tailored to your specific needs.

3. Support Groups: Joining a support group for individuals with gallstones can be a valuable source of information and encouragement. Connecting with others who are going through a similar experience can provide a sense of community and understanding that can help you feel less alone in your recovery journey. Support groups can also be a great place to share tips, resources, and success stories with others who are on the same path.

4. Holistic Practitioners: If you are exploring natural methods for eliminating gallstones, consider working with holistic practitioners such as naturopathic doctors, herbalists, or acupuncturists. These professionals can offer alternative treatments that may complement your overall recovery plan and support your body's natural healing processes.

5. Self-Care Practices: Taking care of yourself is essential during the recovery process. Make time for self-care practices such as meditation, yoga, exercise, and relaxation techniques to reduce stress and promote overall well-being. Remember to listen to your body, prioritize rest, and nourish yourself with a healthy diet and lifestyle choices that support your recovery from gallstones.

By building a strong support system that includes family, friends, healthcare professionals, support groups, holistic practitioners, and self-care practices, you can enhance your chances of successfully eliminating gallstones naturally and promoting overall health and wellness. Remember that recovery is a journey, and having a strong support network can make all the difference in your path to healing.

How To Eliminate Gallstones Naturally

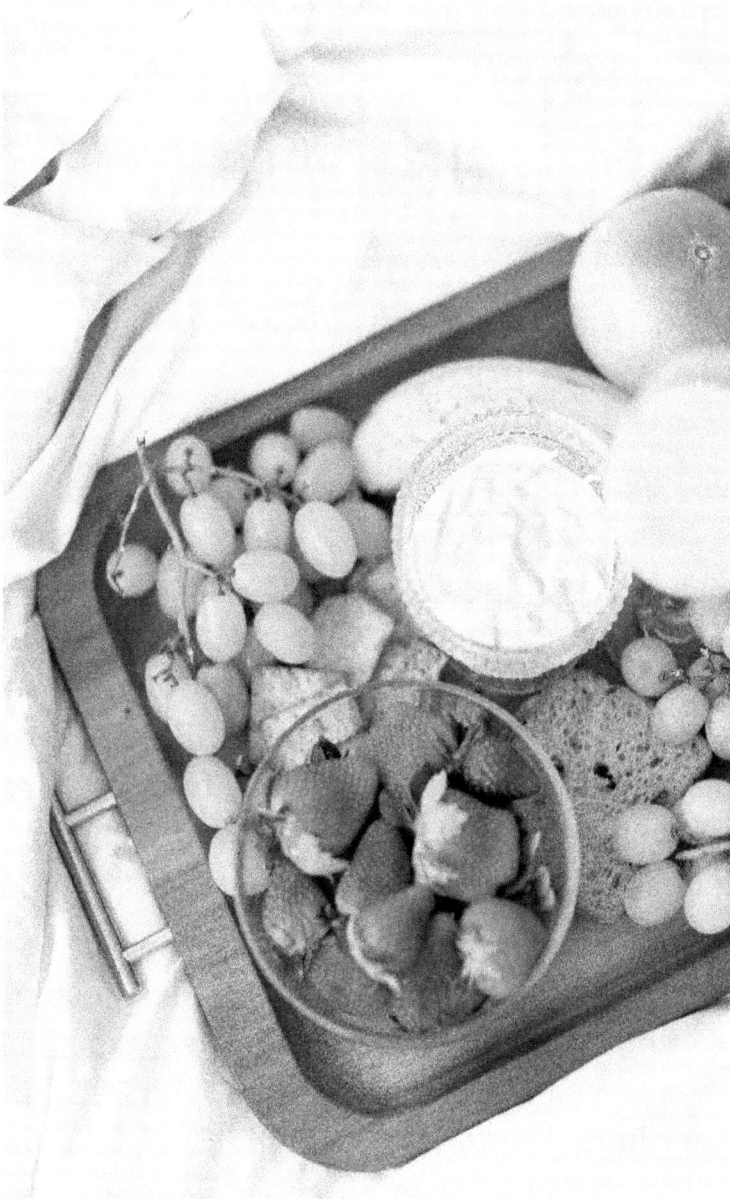

Chapter 9

Success Stories of Gallstone Elimination

Personal Testimonials of Natural Gallstone Elimination

In this subchapter, we will explore personal testimonials from individuals who have successfully eliminated their gallstones using natural methods. These firsthand accounts provide valuable insight and inspiration for those who are seeking an alternative approach to dealing with gallstones. By sharing their experiences, these individuals hope to offer guidance and encouragement to others who are facing similar challenges.

One individual, Sarah, shared her journey of discovering she had gallstones after experiencing severe abdominal pain. Frustrated with the limited options offered by conventional medicine, she turned to natural remedies such as apple cider vinegar and lemon juice to help dissolve her gallstones.

After several weeks of incorporating these remedies into her daily routine, Sarah was amazed to find that her symptoms had significantly improved and her gallstones had disappeared.

Another testimonial comes from John, who had been suffering from gallstone attacks for years. Tired of living in constant pain, he decided to try a holistic approach to eliminate his gallstones. By following a strict diet focused on fresh fruits and vegetables, as well as drinking plenty of water, John was able to gradually dissolve his gallstones over a period of several months. Today, he is symptom-free and grateful for the natural methods that helped him recover.

Rachel, a busy mother of two, also found success in eliminating her gallstones naturally. After experiencing debilitating pain following a fatty meal, she knew she needed to make a change. Through the guidance of a holistic practitioner, Rachel incorporated herbal supplements and liver-cleansing foods into her diet. Within a few months, her gallstones had disappeared, and she was able to enjoy life without the fear of another gallstone attack.

These personal testimonials serve as a reminder that there is hope for those struggling with gallstones. By taking a proactive approach and exploring natural remedies, individuals can find relief and healing without resorting to invasive medical procedures. Whether it's through dietary changes, herbal supplements, or other holistic methods, there are options available for those looking to eliminate gallstones naturally. By learning from the experiences of others, individuals can empower themselves to take control of their health and well-being.

Tips and Advice from Those Who Have Successfully Eliminated Gallstones

In this subchapter, we will explore tips and advice from individuals who have successfully eliminated gallstones using natural methods. These personal stories serve as inspiration and guidance for those who are currently struggling with gallstones and seeking alternative ways to address this common health issue.

One piece of advice that is frequently shared by those who have successfully eliminated gallstones is the importance of maintaining a healthy diet. This includes avoiding high-fat, processed foods and focusing on a diet rich in fruits, vegetables, and whole grains. By making these dietary changes, individuals can reduce the risk of developing new gallstones and promote overall digestive health.

Another tip that is often mentioned is the importance of staying hydrated. Drinking plenty of water throughout the day can help to flush out toxins and prevent the formation of gallstones. Additionally, staying hydrated can support healthy digestion and promote the efficient elimination of waste from the body.

In addition to dietary changes and staying hydrated, many individuals recommend incorporating regular exercise into their routine. Physical activity can help to improve digestion, reduce inflammation, and support overall health. By incorporating a combination of cardiovascular exercise, strength training, and flexibility exercises, individuals can support their body's natural healing processes and reduce the risk of developing new gallstones.

Lastly, individuals who have successfully eliminated gallstones often emphasize the importance of stress management techniques. Stress can have a negative impact on digestive health and contribute to the formation of gallstones. By incorporating relaxation techniques such as deep breathing, meditation, yoga, or massage therapy into their daily routine, individuals can reduce stress levels and support their body's natural healing processes.

By following these tips and advice from those who have successfully eliminated gallstones, individuals can take proactive steps towards improving their health and well-being in a holistic and natural way.

Encouragement for Those on the Path to Recovery

For those who are currently on the path to recovery from gallstones, it is important to remember that you are not alone in this journey. Dealing with gallstones can be a challenging and painful experience, but with the right mindset and support, you can overcome this obstacle.

How To Eliminate Gallstones Naturally

It is crucial to stay positive and focused on your goal of eliminating gallstones naturally. Remember that every step you take towards better health is a step in the right direction.

One of the most important things to remember on your path to recovery is to be patient with yourself. Healing takes time and it is important to give your body the time it needs to heal naturally. Trust in the process and know that with consistency and dedication, you can achieve your goal of eliminating gallstones without the need for surgery or medication. Stay committed to making healthy lifestyle choices and implementing natural remedies that support gallstone elimination.

Surround yourself with a strong support system of family, friends, or a healthcare provider who understands your goals and can offer encouragement along the way. Having a support system can provide you with the motivation and accountability you need to stay on track with your recovery journey. Lean on your support system during challenging times and celebrate your successes together as you progress towards better health.

Remember to prioritize self-care and listen to your body's needs as you navigate the path to recovery. Rest when you need to, nourish your body with healthy foods, and engage in activities that bring you joy and relaxation. Taking care of your physical, mental, and emotional well-being is essential on the road to recovery from gallstones. Practice self-compassion and treat yourself with kindness as you work towards eliminating gallstones naturally.

Lastly, never lose sight of your goal and the progress you have made so far. Celebrate each milestone, no matter how small, and acknowledge the hard work and dedication you have put into your recovery journey. Stay focused on your goal of eliminating gallstones naturally and trust in your body's ability to heal itself. With perseverance, determination, and a positive mindset, you can overcome this obstacle and achieve optimal health and well-being.

How To Eliminate Gallstones Naturally

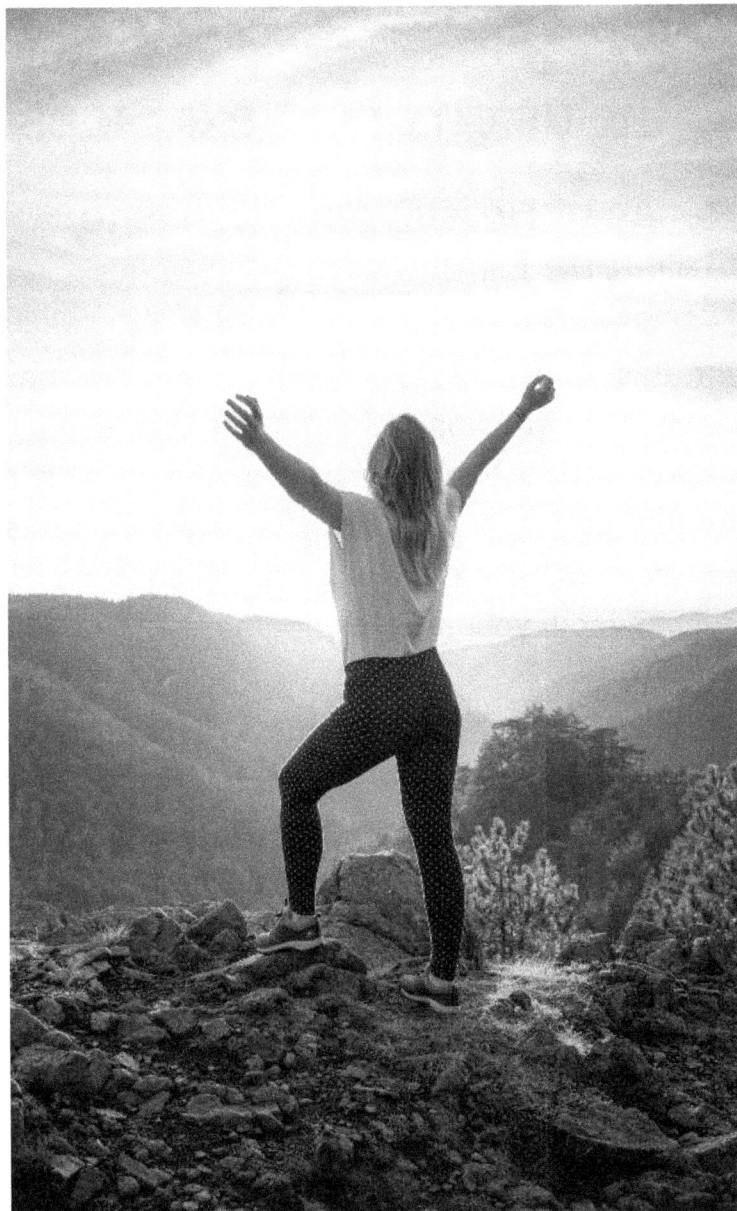

A Holistic Approach to Recovery

Chapter 10

Conclusion and Next Steps

Recap of Holistic Approaches to Gallstone Elimination

In this subchapter, we will recap the holistic approaches to gallstone elimination that have been discussed in this book. For those of you who have gallstones and are looking for natural ways to eliminate them, these holistic approaches can be a game-changer in your recovery journey.

First and foremost, diet plays a crucial role in gallstone elimination. By incorporating foods that are high in fiber, such as fruits, vegetables, and whole grains, you can help prevent the formation of new gallstones and promote the elimination of existing ones. Avoiding high-fat and processed foods is also important, as these can contribute to the development of gallstones.

In addition to diet, staying hydrated is essential for gallstone elimination. Drinking plenty of water throughout the day can help to flush toxins from the body and prevent the buildup of gallstones. Herbal teas, such as dandelion root or milk thistle, can also be beneficial for supporting liver health and aiding in the elimination of gallstones.

Regular exercise is another key component of a holistic approach to gallstone elimination. Physical activity can help improve digestion, promote healthy weight management, and reduce the risk of gallstone formation. Incorporating activities such as walking, yoga, or swimming into your routine can have a positive impact on your overall health and well-being.

Lastly, stress management techniques can be helpful for those dealing with gallstones. Chronic stress can contribute to inflammation in the body, which can exacerbate gallstone symptoms. Practicing mindfulness, deep breathing exercises, or meditation can help reduce stress levels and support the body's natural healing processes.

By incorporating these holistic approaches into your daily routine, you can support your body's natural ability to eliminate gallstones and promote overall health and well-being. Remember, always consult with a healthcare professional before making any significant changes to your diet or lifestyle.

Resources for Further Information and Support

For those who are looking for more information and support on how to eliminate gallstones naturally, there are a variety of resources available to help guide you on your journey to recovery.

Whether you are seeking advice from healthcare professionals, looking for alternative therapies, or simply want to connect with others who are going through a similar experience, there are resources out there to support you every step of the way.

One valuable resource for individuals with gallstones is to seek out guidance from a healthcare provider who specializes in natural or holistic approaches to healing. These practitioners can provide personalized recommendations for dietary changes, supplements, and lifestyle modifications that can help support the body's natural ability to eliminate gallstones. They can also help monitor your progress and adjust your treatment plan as needed.

Another helpful resource for individuals with gallstones is to explore alternative therapies such as acupuncture, herbal medicine, or chiropractic care. These therapies can help address underlying imbalances in the body that may be contributing to the formation of gallstones. By working with experienced practitioners in these modalities, you can uncover new tools and strategies for supporting your body's natural healing process.

In addition to seeking out professional guidance, connecting with others who are going through a similar experience can provide valuable emotional support and encouragement.

Online support groups, forums, and social media communities can be a great way to connect with others who are on a similar healing journey. By sharing your experiences, asking questions, and offering support to others, you can build a network of like-minded individuals who can help you stay motivated and inspired.

Books, articles, and websites dedicated to natural approaches to gallstone elimination can also be valuable resources for individuals looking to learn more about their condition and explore new treatment options. By reading up on the latest research and recommendations from experts in the field, you can gain a deeper understanding of the underlying causes of gallstones and discover new strategies for supporting your body's natural healing process.

Ultimately, the key to successfully eliminating gallstones naturally is to take a comprehensive and holistic approach to your health and well-being. By leveraging the resources available to you, including healthcare providers, alternative therapies, support groups, and educational materials, you can empower yourself to take control of your health and work towards a gallstone-free future.

Committing to a Gallstone-Free Lifestyle

If you have been diagnosed with gallstones, it is important to commit to a gallstone-free lifestyle in order to prevent further complications and improve your overall health. By making small changes to your diet and lifestyle, you can naturally eliminate gallstones and reduce the risk of developing more in the future.

One of the first steps to committing to a gallstone-free lifestyle is to adopt a healthy diet that is rich in fruits, vegetables, whole grains, and lean proteins.

Avoiding high-fat and processed foods is essential, as these can contribute to the formation of gallstones. Instead, focus on incorporating foods that are high in fiber and antioxidants, which can help to break down gallstones and prevent them from forming.

In addition to making changes to your diet, committing to a gallstone-free lifestyle also involves maintaining a healthy weight and staying active. Regular exercise can help to improve digestion, reduce inflammation, and promote gallbladder health. Aim to engage in at least 30 minutes of moderate exercise most days of the week to support your gallstone elimination efforts.

Another important aspect of committing to a gallstone-free lifestyle is staying hydrated. Drinking plenty of water throughout the day can help to flush out toxins and prevent the build-up of gallstones. Aim to drink at least 8-10 glasses of water daily, and consider adding lemon juice or apple cider vinegar to your water for added benefits.

Finally, committing to a gallstone-free lifestyle also involves managing stress and practicing relaxation techniques. Chronic stress can contribute to the formation of gallstones, so it is important to find ways to relax and de-stress on a regular basis. Consider incorporating activities such as yoga, meditation, deep breathing exercises, or spending time in nature to help reduce stress levels and support your gallstone elimination journey.

By making these small but impactful changes to your lifestyle, you can naturally eliminate gallstones and improve your overall health and well-being.

Author Notes & Acknowledgments

First and foremost, I would like to express my deepest gratitude to the people who inspired and supported me throughout the journey of writing this book. This project would not have been possible without their unwavering belief in me and their invaluable contributions.

To my wife, thank you for your constant encouragement and understanding. Your love and support have been my anchor during the challenging times of researching and writing this book. Your belief in my ability to make a difference in people's lives has been my driving force.

I would also like to disclose that this book contains some renewed artificial intelligence-generated content. I really appreciate very recent technological innovation by outstanding scientists and of course our reader's understanding.

Lastly, I want to express my deepest gratitude to the readers of this book. I sincerely hope the strategies and methods outlined within these pages will provide you with the knowledge and tools needed to truly make your life much better. Your commitment to seeking any good solutions and willingness to explore multiple methods is commendable.

Author Bio

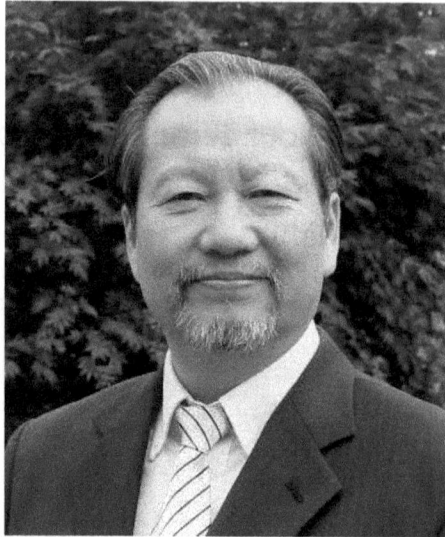

Johnson Wu earned his MD in 1982. With over 40 years of clinical experience, he has worked in hospitals in Zhejiang and Shanghai, China, as well as the Royal Marsden Hospital (part of Imperial College) in London, UK.

Upon the recommendation of Sir Aaron Klug, the president of The Royal Society and a Nobel Prize winner in Chemistry, Dr. Wu was honorably awarded a British Royal Society Fellowship. He has published medical books and articles in seven countries and currently practices medicine in Canada.

www.ingramcontent.com/pod-product-compliance
Lightning Source LLC
Chambersburg PA
CBHW060254030426
42335CB00014B/1688